Table of Contents

GENERAL HISTORY
GENERAL COMPLAINT 6
NEONATAL FEVER 8
PEDIATRIC FEVER 10
FATIGUE 12
WEIGHT LOSS 14
WEIGHT GAIN 16
LUMP/ SWELLING 18
RASH 19
TOCIX INGESTION 21
SUICIDAL ATTEMPT 21
HEADSSS SCREEN 22
INSOMNIA 24
TRAUMA 25
HEAD TRAUMA 26
FOREIGN BODY INGESTION/ ASPIRATION 28
ENT HISTORY
RED EYE 29
SORE THROAT 31
HORSENESS OF VOICE 33
HEARING LOSS 35

TINNITUS	37

CARDIOVASCULAR HISTORY

CHEST PAIN	39
SYNCOPE / LOC	42
PALPITATION	46
EDEMA	48

RESPIRATORY HISTORY

COUGH	50
SHORTNESS OF BREATH	52
STRIDOR	54
HEMOPTYSIS	56

GIT HISTORY

VOMITING	58
HEMATEMESIS	61
DYSPHAGIA	63
JAUNDICE	65
NEONATAL JAUNDICE	67
DIARRHEA	69
CONSTIPATION	72
PEDIATRIC FAILURE TO THRIVE	74
ABDOMINAL PAIN	77
BLOODY STOOL	79

ENDOCRAIN HISTORY

TREMOR	80
DIABETES MELLITUS FOLLOW UP	82

GENITOURIRNARY HISTORY
DYSURIA 83
HEMATURIA 84

ENURESIS IN CHILDREN 86
MENSTRUAL HISTORY 88
SEXUAL HISTORY 88
VAGINAL DISCHARGE 89
PENILE DISCHARGE 90
AMENORRHEA 91
ABNORMAL VAGINAL BLEEDING 94
NEURO HISTORY
ATAXIA 97
SEIZURES 99
HEADACHE 102
MEMORY LOSS 104
MUSKULOSKELETAL HISTORY
JOINT PAIN 106
LOW BACK PAIN 107

CONCISE H&P

Copyright © 2021. All rights reserved to Media Plus. No whole or part of this book can be reproduced in either physical, electronic or any other forms without permission of the author or authorization through payment of appropriate fees.

ISBN 9798561433948

How to structure your assessment?

Identification, PMH, presenting complaint with duration, analysis of presenting complaint with associated symptoms, important related positive and pertinent negative information. PE findings, DDx list.

Example:

John Smith is a 5 yo male who has PMH of asthma, presented with 4 days of cough and 2 days of fever. Fever T max was 103 axillary, intermittently, resolved partially by acetaminophen 5 ml every 4 hr) and cooling measures. Cough started dry and now is productive with thick greenish mucous, with no blood or diurnal variations. Patient's mother denied any shortness of breath, night sweating, appetite or weight changes or sick contacts. For history data and clinical exam findings, most likely diagnosis is URI, asthma execration given his PMH, less likely to be pneumonia given less severe symptoms.

Abbreviations

ABD	Abdominal exam
CVA	Costovertebral Angle
DDx	Differential Diagnosis
EXT	Extremities
EOM	Extraocular Muscles Movement
FH	Family History
GBS	Group B Streptococci infection
GEN	General exam
Hx	History
Meds	Medications
MUSK	Musculoskeletal exam
NEURO	Neuro exam
PMH	Past Medical History
PSH	Past Surgical History
PE	Physical Exam
Sxs	Symptoms
SOB	Shortness of Breath
R	Right
L	Left

GENERAL COMPLAINT

Onset
Constant
Duration / lasts for….
Progression
Frequency
Alleviating factors
Aggravating factors
Associated symptoms
Previous episodes

Past medical History:
Hx of chronic illness:
when diagnosed
Specialist following up
Last follow up
Recent changes
Treatment prescribed
Complications
Hx of hospitalization or ED visit
- Last visit
- Reason
- days admitted
- Any ICU admission
- Intubation subsequent Hx

Past Surgical Hx:
any previous surgery (when, indication, complication)

any complications with general anesthesia in the patient or patient's family (if Preoperative assessment)

Medication Hx:
- Name of drug
- Dose
- Frequency
- Compliance

Family Hx: similar symptoms, FH of chronic illnesses, FH sudden death at young age, FH of genetic diseases

Social Hx:
Living with
Pets
Recent travel
Insurance

FOR PEDIATRIC PATIENTS ask about:

Perinatal History:
Maternal diseases during pregnancy
Infections during pregnancy
Adequate Prenatal care
Place of Delivery
Mood of Delivery
Term/ Preterm   x weeks
Birth Weight
NICU stay, Intubation, other procedures special needs at time of discharge like *(discharge on O2, medication, Tube feeding)*

Nutritional Hx
Feeding type
Breast feeding: # min spent feeding, frequency
Formula: Name, Amount, Frequency, Preparation
Cow milk: oz per day
Other food: table food, baby food, any dietary restrictions

Developmental Millstones *(according to age)*

NEONATAL FEVER

Duration
Mode of measurement axillary, oral, rectal, tympanic, Subjective (by touch)
Highest temperature
Fever pattern continuous, intermittent or remittent, undulant
Cooling measures
Associated Symptoms:
- Fussiness, irritability, lethargy
- Decrease PO intake
- Nasal congestion, Rhinorrhea
- Cough, Difficulty breathing
- Vomiting, Diarrhea
- Skin Rash
- Seizures
- Hematuria
- Joint Swelling

Perinatal Hx
Prenatal care
Perinatal maternal infections
- Oral / genital ulcers or lesions
- Fever during pregnancy
- Rash during pregnancy
- GBS status

Immunization:
HX of Recent Vaccination

Meds Hx: (name, dose, indication, compliance)

Family History:
Sick Contact

Social Hx:
Attend daycare
Hx of Recent Travel

PERTIENT PHYSICAL EXAM

Check Vitals: Temperature, HR, RR, BP

Perform complete physical exam to look for focus of infection

GEN: Toxic, ill- appearing, lethargic, irritable
EYE: eye discharge, conjunctivitis, Fundus exam for chorioretinitis (TORCH infection)
HEAD: Microcephaly, bulging AF
SKIN: Rash, petechia
LUNGS: decrease AE, wheeze or crackles
ABD: Hepatosplenomegaly (TORCH infection)

DIFFERENTIAL DIAGNOSIS

Infectious causes (Viral, Bacterial, Rickettsia, Fungal, Parasitic)
- Neonatal Sepsis
- Pneumonia
- Meningitis
- Urinary tract infection
- Septic arthritis, osteomyelitis
- Congenital infections TORCH
- Upper respiratory tract infection

Non-Infectious causes
- Oncological
e.g. Leukemia, Lymphoma, Solid tumors
- Drug induced
e.g. Phenytoin, Carbamazepine, Isoniazid

PEDIATRIC FEVER

Onset
Duration
Mode of measurement
Highest temperature
Fever pattern continuous, intermittent or remittent, undulant
Use of antipyretic: Dose, Last dose, Dose frequency every …. Hours
Effect of Antipyretic (temperature is back to normal, lower T but never normal)
Associated Symptoms:
– Fussiness, Ear tugging, ear pain
– Nasal congestion, Rhinorrhea
– Facial tenderness, Headache
– Pink eye, Eye pain or swelling
– Cough, Difficulty breathing
– Skin Rash
– Sore throat, Neck swelling, painful swallowing
– SOB, Chest pain
– Photophobia, Neck Rigidity
– Delirium, Seizures
– Vomiting, Diarrhea
– Dysuria +/- Hematuria
– Joint pain, Joint Swelling
– Night sweating, Wt or appetite Loss

Meds:
Recent use of antibiotic or other meds
(Name, reason, dose, duration taken)

Immunization
Immunized or not
Up to date vaccination
HX of Recent Vaccination

Allergy: any known drug allergies?

FH: Similar sxs in family

Social Hx:
daycare attendance
Animal contact
unpasteurized milk, raw meat, fish, well-water
Hx of Recent Travel

PERTIENT PHYSICAL EXAM

Check Vitals: Temperature, HR, RR, BP
Perform complete physical exam to look for a focus of infection

DIFFERENTIAL DIAGNOSIS

Infectious causes (Viral, Bacterial, Rickettsial, Fungal, Parasitic)
- Upper respiratory tract infection URI
- Pneumonia
- Pharyngitis, Tonsillitis
- Dental, Peritonsillar or Retropharyngeal Abscesses
- Sinusitis
- Acute otitis media, Acute otitis externa
- Orbital retroorbital abscesses
- Brain abscess, Meningitis, encephalitis
- Acute gastroenteritis, Cholecystitis, pancreatitis
- Urinary tract infection (UTI)
- Pelvic inflammatory disease, STI
- Septic arthritis, osteomyelitis
- TB, Malaria

Non-Infectious causes
- Oncological e.g. Leukemia, Lymphoma, HLH, Solid tumors
- Autoimmune e.g. SLE, JIA, IBD, Kawasaki disease
- Endocrine e.g. Hyperthyroidism, thyrotoxicosis, DI
- Drug induced e.g. Phenytoin, Carbamazepine, Isoniazid ….ect
- Fever of unknown origin

FATIGUE

Duration
Course: worsening, Constant
Diurnal variation
Sleep hygiene
Caffeine intake
Snoring/ Sleep apnea
Daytime sleepiness
Early morning waking
Life Stressors/ Difficulty concentrating
Changes in living circumstances
Long working hours
Comprehensive Review of Systems
- Fever, chills, weight loss or gain, appetite changes, night sweats
- Red eye, visual problems
- ear pain, congestion, sore throat
- Cough, SOB
- N/V/D, constipation, rectal bleeding
- Dysuria, hematuria, genital discharge
- excessive thirst, excessive hunger, cold intolerance
- Rash, Petechia, bruises, bleeding, swollen glands
- Muscle pain, joint pain, joint swelling, joint stiffness
- Seizures, LOC, numbness, weakness
- Depressed mood, anxiety

PMH: any chronic disease

Meds Hx: current medications (name, dose, indication, compliance)

FH: FH of malignancy, Autoimmune diseases or any other diseases run in the family

Social Hx: lives with, smoking, drug abuse *(HEADSSS screening, see page 22).*
Diet: Vegetarian?
Recent travel

PERTIENT PHYSICAL EXAM

Check Vital sings

GEN: Body built, muscle wasting, cold intolerance

NECK: Thyroid exam, lymph nodes

CVS: murmur, gallop

RESP: cough, hemoptysis, tachypnea, retraction, wheeze, crackles

ABD: organomegaly or masses

HEME: Pallor, bruises

NEURO: muscle weakness, decrease reflexes

PSYCH: Flat effect, depressed mood, poor eye contact, muffled voice

DIFFERENTIAL DIAGNOSIS

- Hypothyroidism
- Sleep Apnea
- MDD
- Generalized anxiety disorders
- Anemia
- Malignancy
- DM/ DI
- Myasthenia Gravis
- Myopathies
- Rheumatological diseases
- hypercalcemia
- Renal Failure
- Heart failure

WEIGHT LOSS

Duration
How did you know? Scale/ *Cloths size*
How many kg / lb lost over what duration?
Intentional or not?
Personal body image
Recent change in diet
Detailed diet Hx

- how many meals/day
- Meal size
- How many snakes/day
- Type of food
- Any dietary restriction

Recent change in appetite
Exercise habits
Associated Sxs
- fever, night sweats
- Chronic cough, SOB
- Palpitations
- Heat intolerance
- Tremor, neck mass
- skin pigmentation
- Polydipsia/polyuria
- Nausea/ vomiting
- Food regurgitation / heartburn
- Dysphagia
- Jaundice (yellow skin & sclera)
- Abdominal distension/ Bloating
- Diarrhea, greasy stools
- Bloody stool
- Last menstrual period
- Secondary amenorrhea

PMH: Any chronic illness
Meds Hx: Laxative or diuretic use, other meds (name, dose, indication, compliance)
Family Hx: Hx of malignancy in family, IBD, endocrinopathies
Social Hx:
Who patient lives with, Access to /Availability of food
Sexual Hx, Alcohol intake or illicit drug use

PERTIENT PHYSICAL EXAM

Vitals: BP, RR, HR, T (bradycardia & hypothermia in anorexia nervosa), Orthostatic vitals (Addison dz, dehydration)
Anthropometrics: Wt, Ht, Centiles *(for children)*, BMI
General: pallor, cachexic
Mouth: oral ulcers
CVS: tachycardia, arrhythmia
Lung: decrease breath sounds, crackles, wheeze
Abd: Abdominal distension, hepatosplenomegaly, anal lesions
Skin: hyperpigmentation, rash
MSK: clubbing, muscle wasting, joint swelling, tremors

DIFFERENTIAL DIAGNOSIS

Decrease caloric intake

- Anorexia nervosa & other eating disorders
- Swallowing disorders e.g. achalasia, esophageal tumors
- alcoholism
- Abuse/ neglect & poverty
- Voluntary wt loss

Absorption problems

- CF
- Celiac disease
- Inflammatory bowel disease
- Malabsorption syndromes
- **Increased metabolism**
- Hyperthyroidism
- Stress
- Increased physical activity
- Malignancy
- Endocrinopathies: DM, DI, , Addison's disease
- Chronic diseases

- Infections: chronic (TB, HIV, bacterial, fungal, parasites) or severe acute infection/ illnesses

Iatrogenic
Laxative, thyroxine & diuretic abuse

WEIGHT GAIN

Duration
How did you know? Scale/ Cloths size
How many kg / lb gained over what duration
Recent change in diet
Recent change in physical activity
Detailed diet Hx
- how many meals/day
- Meal size
- How many snakes/da
- Type of food
- Frequency of eating fast food
- Bing eating

Associated Sxs
- Depressed mood
- Recent stress
- Fatigue
- Decrease urine output
- Jaundice (yellow skin & sclera)
- Orthopnea/ exertional dyspnea
- Cold intolerance
- Hair / eyebrows thinning
- Increase facial hair in females
- Acne
- Menstrual irregularity
- Last menstrual period
- Decrease libido
- Hot flushes
- Polydipsia, polyurea

PMH: Any chronic or psychiatric illnesses
PSH: any previous surgeries

Meds Hx: Steroids, Antidepressant, Antipsychotics, anticonvulsants, oral Contraceptives
Other medications (name, dose, indication, compliance)

Family Hx: FH of obesity, endocrinopathies

Social Hx: Recently stopped smoking, daily alcohol intake

PERTIENT PHYSICAL EXAM

Vital sings: BP, RR, HR, T
Parameters: Wt, Ht, Centiles (child) BMI
  General: Dysmorphic features, developmental delay, signs of resp. distress, flat affect, depressed mood.
Eye: papilledema
Mouth: tonsillar hypertrophy
Neck: Thyroid
CVS: murmur, gallop, LLE, weak pulses
Lungs: retractions, air entry, crackles
Abd: ascites, organomegaly
Genitalia: tanner stage
Skin: acanthosis nigricans, Hirsutism, acne, stria, jaundice, palmer erythema, spider nevi

Medications: chronic use of

- Steroids
- Antidepressant SSRI, TCA, amitriptyline
- Antipsychotics
- Anticonvulsants, valproate
- oral Contraceptive contains progesterone

Recent smoking cessation

DIFFERENTIAL DIAGNOSIS

Increase caloric intake

Decrease caloric consumption, less exercise

Fluid retention

- Congestive heart failure
- Hepatic failure
- Renal failure

Endocrinopathies

- Hypothyroidism
- Cushing syndrome
- Hyperinsulinemia
- Polycystic ovary disease
- Hypogonadism
- Syndromes associated with Obesity

Pregnancy

LUMP/ SWELLING

Location
Duration
Number if >1
Distribution if >1
Caused by

- Hx of trauma
- Insect bite
- others

Course: worsening, Constant
Hx of Trauma
Previous similar lump
Associated Sxs

- fever
- pain (ask about SOCRATES)
- itchiness
- burning sensation
- swelling
- skin changes
- discharge
- bleeding

PMH: any chronic illnesses

PSH: any previous surgery

Meds Hx: current medications (name, dose, indication, compliance)

Vaccination Hx: recent vaccination

Family Hx: family members with similar sxs?

Social Hx: recent travel, pet or wild animal contact

EXAMINING SWELLING/LUMP
Site
Size
Shape
Skin changes
Surface
Tenderness
Consistency
Fluctuance
Mobility
Transillumination
Pulsation
Bruit

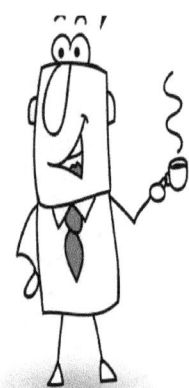

RASH

Duration
Location: Generalized/ localized to
Progression: started at .. then moved to...
Pattern of distribution: annular, dermatomal...
Color & any color changes
Presence of 2ry lesion: scales, crust..
Itchy or not
Painful or not
Hx of use of contact with new products or cloths
Associated sxs
- Fever
- Cough
- Congestion
- Conjunctivitis
- Sore throat
- Joint swelling

PMH: skin disorders, other chronic conditions

PSH: any previous surgeries

Meds Hx: current medication (name, dose, indication, compliance)

Vaccination Hx: Hx of recent vaccination

Allergy: allergy to food or medications
Hx of anaphylaxis or allergic rash

Family Hx: similar sxs in the family, inherited skin disorders

Social Hx:
Pets at home
Recent animal contact
Recent travel
Sexual Hx (*acquired immunodeficiency*)

PERTIENT PHYSICAL EXAM

Perform Complete PE
Examine the whole skin, nails & mucous membranes

Description of Rash

1. **Location:** Localized to …/ generalized
2. **Involved palms & soles or not**
3. **Color:**
4. **Lesion type:**
   - **1ry lesions:**
   Macule, papule, nodule, vesicle, bullae, pustule, burrow, telangiectasia
   - **2ry lesions:**
   Scales, crust, atrophic, ulcer, fissure, petechia, purpura, ecchymosis
5. **Lesions arrangement:** Annular, dermatomal, follicular, reticular, multiform, morbilliform
6. **Texture:** smooth, rough, lichenification, indurated, sand & pepper like, …

If non- specific lesions include above plus:

shape of lesion, flat or raised, margins and consistency

TOXIC INGESTION

Time of ingestion
What was ingested?
Quantity ingested
What is in the home medicine cabinet
(Possible co-ingestions)
Route of ingestion
Witnessed or not
Reason of ingestion intentional/ not
Suicidal attempt
Previous episodes
Associated Sxs
- Vomiting
- LOC
- Seizures

PMH: any chronic illness including psychiatric disorders
PSH: any previous surgeries
Meds Hx: current medication

Social Hx: HEADSSS screen *(see next page 22)*

Suicidal Attempt

Time
Method
If pills: #, dose strength mg/ pill, extended release, Co-ingestions
If other plans, what happened
Witnessed or not
Motive for suicide
Was attempt planned or impulsive
Continued desire to commit suicide
Is there a definite plan?

PMH: Hx of psychiatric disorders, Previous suicide attempts or threats.
Meds:
Family History: Depression, suicide, psychiatric disorders
Social History: who you live with, social support, **HEADSSS screen** *(see page22)*

HEADSSS Screen

Home:

- Who do you live with?
- Any recent changes at home
- Relationship with partner, parents, siblings
- Do you feel safe at home? If not, Why?

Education/ Employment

- School grade/field of study, performance
- Any recent changes at school?
- bullying at school/ work
- Favorite/ unfavorite subjects
- Any current employment
- Relationship to co-workers/ teachers/ peers

Activities:

- What do you do for fun?
- Hoppies/ Extracurricular activities
- Screen time?

Drugs/ Behavior

- Use of cigarette smoking/ vaping
- Use of alcohol or illicit drugs
    - Amount
    - Frequency
- Use of seatbelt
- Hx of arrest/ incarceration/ crime

Sleep

- What time you go to bed?
- How many hours of sleep/day?
- Frequent waking at night
- Early morning waking

Sexuality:

- Orientation
- # of current partners?
- of partners over last year?
- Use of contraception/Barriers
- Hx of STIs/ Treatment
- Hx of abortion or pregnancy

Suicide/ Depression:

- Appetite changes
- Loss of interest in doing your favorite activities.
- Feeling of isolation/ withdrawal
- Feeling hopeless or helpless
- Any recent stressor in your life
- Hx or current suicidal or homicidal ideation
- If yes, Do you have a definitive plan?
- Guns at home? Locked or not
- Hx of suicidal attempts in the past
- Hx of psychiatric disorders or counseling

PERTIENT PHYSICAL EXAM

Check vital signs & O2 sat

GEN: personal hygiene, signs of trauma, built,

EYE: Pupils size (miosis or mydriasis), nystagmus

SKIN: flushed, dry, diaphoretic, cyanosis

NEURO: GCS, mental status, tone, reflexes, gait

PSYCH: look for following signs

Affect: flat, anxious, tearful, depressed, paranoid, hostile, non-communicative

Behavior: cooperative, aggressive, relaxed, combative, belligerent

Judgement: Impaired, abnormal thoughts

Thoughts: delusional, obsessive, hallucinating, flight of ideas

INSOMNIA

Duration
How many hrs you sleep a day?
Interrupted sleep at night
Restless sleep at night
Early morning waking
When you wake in the morning do you feel you are tired or not?
snoring?
Observed apnea during sleeping
Prefers use >1 pillow
Headache during daytime
Daytime sleepiness
Learning difficulties in school/ difficulty focusing on work

Comprehensive Review of Systems

- Fever, chills, weight loss or gain, appetite changes, night sweats
- Visual problems
- Congestion, sore throat
- Cough, SOB
- N/V/D, constipation, rectal bleeding
- Dysuria, hematuria, genital discharge
- excessive thirst, excessive hunger, cold intolerance
- Rash, Petechia, spontaneous bruises or bleeding, swollen glands
- Muscle pain, joint pain, joint swelling, stiffness
- Seizures, LOC, numbness, weakness
- Depressed mood, anxiety

PMH: any chronic illnesses

PSH: any previous surgeries

Meds Hx: current medication (name, dose, indication, compliance)

Family Hx: any diseases run in the family

Social Hx: HEADSSS screen *(see page 22)*

TRAUMA/ MVA

Time of trauma
Place where accident happened
How transported to hospital
Mechanism of injury
Speed of vehicle
Side of impact
Use of Protective gears (seatbelt or helmet)
Ejected from vehicle?
Death of other passengers
Last meal
Other sxs
- LOC, how long
- Seizures
- Bleeding
- Extremities deformities
- Abdominal pain
- Vomiting
- Breathing problems
- Visual changes
- Clear fluid or blood coming from nose or ear

PMH: bleeding disorders, other chronic medical conditions

PSH: previous surgeries

Meds Hx: anticoagulants, current medications (name, dose, indication, compliance)

Vaccination Hx: last Tetanus vaccine

Allergy: allergy to any medications

Family Hx:

Social Hx: suspected alcohol or substance intoxication
Social circumstance for suspected abuse or neglect

HEAD TRAUMA

Time of Accident
Witnessed or not
Place where accident happened
Mechanism of injury
Height
If fall from stairs: # of stairs
Surface of impact (Tiled floor, Carpeted floor..)
Side of impact
Use of Protective gears (seatbelt or helmet)
Last meal

Other sxs
- LOC, how long
- Vomiting
- Headache
- Seizures
- Ataxia
- Sleepy/ Lethargy
- Amnesia
- Behavioral changes
- Bleeding
- Visual changes
- Clear fluid or blood coming from nose or ear

PMH: bleeding disorders, other chronic medical conditions

PSH: previous surgeries, Hx anesthesia complications

Meds Hx: anticoagulants, current medications (name, dose, indication, compliance)

Vaccination Hx:

Allergy:

Social Hx: suspected alcohol or substance intoxication
Social circumstance for suspected abuse or neglect

Pediatric Head Injury
Use PECARN Algorithm to assess the severity of traumatic brain injury and the indications for Head CT & neurosurgical interventions

- Age > or < 2 years of age
- Mechanism of injury
  (If fall: height > 5 ft for children > 2 years of age or > 3 ft for children < 2 years of age)
- LOC >5 Sec
- Vomiting > x2
- Behavioral changes/headache / neurological deficits
- GCS <15
- palpable skull # or occipital or temporal scalp hematoma

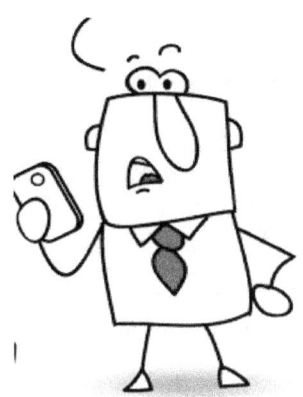

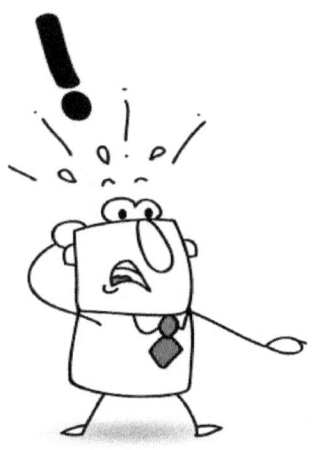

Signs of Basilar Skull Fracture
- Periorbital bruising (Raccoon eyes)
- Retro-auricular bruising (Battle's sign)
- Hemotympanum
- CSF otorrhea
- CSF rhinorrhea

FOREIGN BODY INGESION/ ASPIRATION

Object ingested
Time of ingestion
Witnessed or not
Sudden cough, chocking
Associated sxs
- Stridor
- SOB/ wheezing
- Chest pain
- Drooling/ gagging
- FB sensation
- Sore throat
- painful swallowing
- Refusal to eat
- Vomiting
- Abd pain
- Abd distension
- Bloody stool

Ear foreign body
- Ear pain
- Hearing loss
- Ear discharge
- Ear bleed
- Foul smelling odor from ear

PMH: hx of intellectual disabilities or developmental delay, psychiatric disorders, hx of chronic illnesses

PSH: any previous surgery, when, indication, complications, Hx of complications from anesthesia

Meds Hx: any current medications (name, dose, indication, compliance)

Allergy: any drug or food allergies

Family Hx:

Social Hx:

RED EYE

Duration
Side: R / L
Course: worsening, Constant
Preceding URI
Hx of foreign body
Hx of chemical exposure
Hx of Trauma
Wearing Contacts?
Previous episodes
Associated Sxs
- Eye swelling
- Eye discharge (*Amount, Color*)
- Itchiness
- Tearing
- Burning sensation
- Photophobia
- Painful eye movement
- Restricted eye movement
- Visual changes
- Headache
- Fever
- Rash
- Cough/ congestion/ rhinorrhea

Maternal Hx of STIs *(For neonates)*

PMH: hx of chronic illnesses

PSH: any previous surgery, when, indication, complications

Meds Hx: name, dose, indication, compliance

Vaccination Hx: up to date or not

Allergy: any drug or food allergies

Family Hx: similar condition in family members

Social Hx: recent travel, animal contact

PERTIENT PHYSICAL EXAM

Check vital signs

Perform complete exam with focus on eyes

Eye exam

- inspect eyelid, lashes, conjunctiva *(bulbar, palpebral)* for or erythema or swelling, proptosis or discharge
- visual acuity
- EOM
- Pupils: shape, size, light reaction, hyphemia *(blood in ant. Chamber)*
- fundus

DIFFERENTIAL DIAGNOSIS

- Allergic conjunctivitis
- Viral conjunctivitis
- Bacterial conjunctivitis
- Corneal abrasions (trauma)
- Preseptal orbital cellulitis
- Orbital cellulitis
- Endophthalmitis
- Keratitis / Uveitis/ Episcleritis/ Iritis
- Glaucoma
- Conjunctivitis associated with Systemic illnesses like viral syndrome, rheumatological diseases, Kawasaki disease

Causes of neonatal conjunctivitis (ophthalmia Neonatorum)

- Chemical conjunctivitis (1st day due to topical erythromycin ointment)
- Gonorrheal conjunctivitis (2-5 days after birth)
- Chlamydial conjunctivitis (>5 days after birth)
- Birth Trauma
- Congenital glaucoma

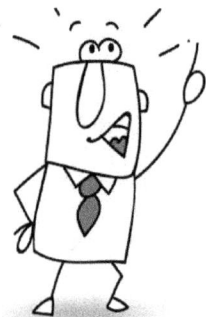

SORE THEOAT

Duration
Is pain always present or only on swallowing?
Severity 1-10
Course: worsening, constant
Location: R, L
Aggravating factors: speaking, coughing, swallowing
Relieving factors: pain meds, ..
Hx of foreign body or trauma
Inhalational/chemical exposure
Associated sxs

- Fever
- Neck pain/ neck swelling
- Nasal congestion/discharge
- Cough
- SOB
- Noisy breathing
- Voice changes
- Ear pain
- Red eyes
- Rash
- Headache
- Abdominal pain
- Appetite / Wt loss

PMH: Hx of streptococcal pharyngitis, scarlet fever, rheumatic fever, immunocompromised

PSH: Any previous surgeries

Meds Hx: any current medications

Allergy:

Family Hx: FH of similar sxs, any family member recently diagnosed with Strep pharyngitis

Social Hx: sexual Hx, recent travel

PERTIENT PHYSICAL EXAM

Check Vital sings & O2 saturation

GEN: Ill /Toxic, sings of acute distress, drooling, muffled voice

EYE: conjunctivitis *(adenovirus)*

MOUTH: Trismus, pharyngeal erythema, petechiae, vesicles or ulcerations (HPV, Coxsackie virus), tonsillar enlargement or exudates, deviated uvula, cobblestoning *(allergic rhinitis)*

NECK: ant/post. tender cervical lymphadenopathy, neck swelling or erythema

RESP: inspiratory stridor, retractions, decreased breath sounds

ABD: hepatosplenomegaly *(EBV, CMV)*

SKIN: rash, cyanosis

DIFFERENTIAL DIAGNOSIS

- Viral pharyngitis including EBV, HSV
- Bacterial pharyngitis including Group A strep & gonococcal pharyngitis
- Tonsillitis
- Acute epiglottitis
- Vincent angina
- Peritonsillar abscess
- Retropharyngeal abscess
- Allergic rhinitis
- Acute thyroiditis
- Scarlet fever
- Kawasaki disease
- Throat FB

HOARSNESS OF VOICE

Onset: sudden, gradual
Duration
Overuse of voice
Painful or painless
Progression
Previous episodes
Associated sxs
- Neck swelling
- Heartburn
- Fever
- Chills
- Chronic cough
- Hemoptysis
- Neck mass
- Appetite / Wt loss
- Night sweats
- Recent URI

PMH: Hx of Stroke, Hx of chronic GERD, hypothyroid, or any other chronic diseases
Hx of intubation

PSH: Any hx of thyroid or cardiothoracic surgeries

Meds Hx: any current medication

Immunization: As per mother (*if you did not see vaccination record*) up to date, including annual flu vaccine

Allergy: any known allergies?

Family Hx: similar sxs in your family

Social Hx:
Occupation
Smoking
alcohol abuse
Recent travel

PERTIENT PHYSICAL EXAM

Perform complete physical exam

Laryngoscope exam required in those patients if chronic symptoms >3 weeks

DIFFERENTIAL DIAGNOSIS

Infectious laryngitis

Inflammation/ VC Edema

- Voice overuse
- GERD
- Allergies
- Smoking
- Trauma during intubation or endoscopy

Neoplasms

- Pharyngeal polyps, nodule or carcinoma

Neurological

- Recurrent Laryngeal Never palsy due to external compression or Trauma during thyroid or thoracic surgeries
- Degenerative diseases like Parkinsonism, amyloidosis

Miscellaneous

- Inhaled steroids
- Hypothyroidism
- Acromegaly

HEARING LOSS

Duration
Which side?
Onset sudden / gradual
Course
High- or low-pitched sounds
Exposure to loud noise
Object inserted in the ear
Hx of ear trauma
Hx of recurrent otitis media
Associated sxs:
- Ear pain
- Ear discharge
- Fever
- Ringing in the ears
- Sense of ear fullness
- Vertigo/ Dizziness
- Headache
- Facial weakness or numbness
- Double vision

PMH: DM, Autoimmune diseases, Stroke, MS, Renal failure, Syphilis

PSH: any previous surgeries

Meds: ASA or other NSAID, loop diuretics, aminoglycosides, Cisplatin, minocycline others

Family Hx: hearing loss running in family or kidney problems

Social Hx Occupation (*noise exposure*)
Hobbies e.g. scoba diving, flying *(Barotrauma)*
Sexual Hx
Smoking, alcohol intake, illicit drugs abuse

PERTIENT PHYSICAL EXAM

Eye: nystagmus, EOM, pupils
Ear exam: ear shape, external canal, drums
Weber & Rinne Tests
Complete neuro exam: including cranial nerves, cerebellar signs and gait
Skin: hyperpigmented café au late spots, neurofibromas, facial hemangiomas, ash leaf nodules

DIFFERENTIAL DIAGNOSIS

Conductive hearing loss

- External Auditory canal obstruction
- (e.g. Cerumen impaction, Foreign body, Cholesteatoma, congenital or acquired neoplasms, congenital or acquired stenosis or atresia, edema of auditory canal from severe Otitis exaterna)
- Trauma
- Middle ear effusion
- Otosclerosis
- Drum perforation
- Barotrauma

Sensorineural hearing loss

- Noise induced
- Meniere's disease
- Presbycusis *(old patients)*
- Ototoxic medications induced
- Inner ear or skll-base neoplasms e.g. Acoustic Neuroma, schwannoma, meningioma
- Infections e.g. TORCH infection in newborns, syphilis, viral labyrinthitis, meningitis
- Multiple sclerosis

TINNITUS

Duration
Side: R or L Ear
Character blowing, clicking
Course: worsening, constant
Frequency: intermittent, static
Previous episodes
Relieving or alleviating factors
Does it pulse with heartbeat?
Ear trauma
Recent Hx of head trauma
Exposure to loud noise
Associated Sxs

- Vertigo
- Nausea/ vomiting
- Hearing loss
- Fever
- Nasal congestion

PMH:

PSH: any previous surgeries

Meds Hx: Aspirin, current medication including OTC or supplements

Allergy:

Family Hx: FH of similar sxs, FH of hearing loss or with hearing aids

Social Hx:

PERTIENT PHYSICAL EXAM

Check vital signs

Eye: nystagmus, EOM, pupils, pallor

Ear exam: ear canals for cerumen impaction, drums

Weber & Rinne Tests

Complete neuro exam: including cranial nerves, Babinski sign, cerebellar signs and gait

Skin: hyperpigmented café au late spots, neurofibromas, facial hemangiomas, ash leaf nodules (*risk for acoustic neuroma*)

DIFFERENTIAL DIAGNOSIS

- Meniere's disease
- Otosclerosis
- Labyrinthitis
- Benign Intracranial hypertension
- Acoustic neuroma
- Cerebellopontine angle tumors
- Vascular tumors, AVM
- Noise-induced tinnitus
- Salicylate toxicity
- Multiple sclerosis
- High cardiac output status like in anemia, pregnancy, or fever

CHEST PAIN

Location
Duration
Onset: sudden, gradual
Quality: sharp, stabbing, pressure like, burning
Course: worsening, constant, improving
Frequency intermittent, static
How long it lasts?
Radiation
Severity 1-10
Previous episodes
Happened at Rest
Hx of chest trauma
Aggravating factors

- Exercise
- Eating
- Emotional stress
- Deep breathing or coughing
- Lying down
- Certain position

Relieving factors

Associated Sxs

- Fever
- Sweating
- SOB
- Syncope
- Palpitation
- Cough
- Cyanosis
- Orthopnea
- Lower extremities swelling
- Wt or appetite Loss
- Wheeze

PMH:
Hx of murmur or congenital heart disease
Hx of DM, hypertension, hyperlipidemia or coronary artery disease
Hx of peptic ulcers, reflux ….

PSH: Any Previous surgeries

Meds Hx: any medications including OTC

Vaccination Hx:

Allergy:

Family Hx:
FH of sudden death
Hx of cardiac disease running in the family
FH of premature CAD

Social Hx:
Diet & lifestyle
Recent travel
Cocaine abuse, other illicit drugs abuse or Smoking

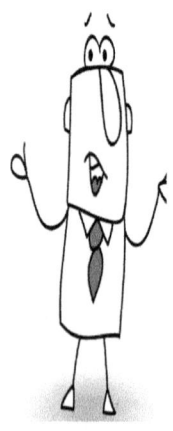

RED FLAGS FOR SERIOUS CHEST PAIN
Sudden onset
Severe pain
Pain on exercise
With SOB
With syncope
With vomiting
Hemodynamically unstable patient *(tachycardia, hypotension, tachypnea, cyanosis)*
Murmur, gallop or pericardial rub on exam

PERTIENT PHYSICAL EXAM

Check Vitals: T, HR, RR, BP

APPERANCE: Ill /Toxic, Built, dysmorphism *(syndromes associated with CHD)*, sings of acute distress

HANDS: perfusion, cyanosis, nails for clubbing and splinter hemorrhage, Palmer creases for pallor, Xanthoma

CHEST: Tenderness at cost sternal junction, subcutaneous emphysema, Retractions, Breath sounds, Crackles or wheeze

BREAST: asymmetry, enlargement, tenderness

CVS: Regular/ irregular rhythm & rate, murmur (location, systolic/ diastolic, intensity, grade), rub, Peripheral pulses, LLE

ABD: abdominal dissension, hepatomegaly

SKIN: bruises *(trauma)*

DIFFERENTIAL DIAGNOSIS

Cardiac

- Pericarditis
- Myocarditis
- Myocardial infarction
- Dysrhythmias (SVT, VT)
- Coronary artery spams
- Hypertrophic cardiomyopathy
- Aortic dissection
- Mitral valve prolapse
- Kawasaki disease

Musculoskeletal

- Costochondritis
- Chest wall strain
- Chest trauma

Respiratory

- Pulmonary embolism
- Asthma
- Pneumonia
- Pneumothorax
- Pneumomediastinum
- Pleuritis
- Severe pulmonary hypertension

Gastrointestinal

- GERD
- Esophageal spasms
- Esophagitis
- Gastritis
- Peptic ulcer
- Pancreatitis
- Cholecystitis

Others

- Cocaine toxicity
- Herpes zoster
- Anxiety

SYNCOPE/ LOSS OF CONSCIOUSNESS

When it happened?
Duration of LOC
Previous episodes
Witnessed or not

i-Pre-syncopal

When it happened?
What patient was doing prior to episode?
- Standing from sitting
- Standing for long time
- Syncope during exercise
- Syncope after exercise
- Strong emotion
- Coughing or straining
- Abrupt neck movement

Who witnessed the event?
Any presyncope sxs?
- Nausea/Vomiting
- Diarrhea
- Poor Fluid intake
- Sweating
- Lightheaded
- Palpitation
- Flushing
- SOB
- Weakness
- auditory or visual changes

ii-Syncopal
- Abnormal body movement or position
- Abnormal eye movement
- Tongue biting
- Incontinences (Bladder/Bowel)

iii-Post-Syncopal
- Does patient remember any details?
- Weakness
- Speech difficulty
- Amnesia
- Confusion

PMH
Arrythmias, Congenital Heart Disease, Seizure disorders, Migraine, DM (Hypo or hyperglycemia, autonomic neuropathy), Adrenal insufficiency
Other chronic diseases

PSH: Any previous surgery, when, indication, complications

Meds Hx:
B-Blockers, Diuretics, Vasodilators, CCB, Clonidine, sedative, anticonvulsants any other medications

FH:
Syncope, sudden death, seizures, cardiac disease, arrythmias, migraine
any family member with pacemaker

Social Hx:
Who do you live with?
Diet & lifestyle
Recent travel
Alcohol or illicit drugs abuse
Smoking

PERTIENT PHYSICAL EXAM FOR SYNCOPE

Check vitals Pulse, BP from both arms, and O2 saturation

orthostatic pulse and BP

GEN: signs of distress, hydration status, perfusion

FUNDSCOPY: papilledema

CVS: Precordial thrill, Heart sounds, murmur, gallop, rub

Carotid bruits, peripheral pulses

NEURO complete neurological exam

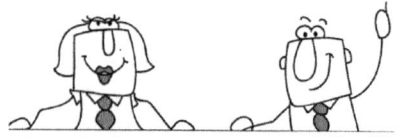

WHEN TO REFERER SYNCOPE TO CARDIOLOGIST?

- √ Syncope during exercise
- √ Syncope without warning signs (likely arrythmia)
- √ Syncope with positive FH of sudden cardiac death or arrythmias like WPW syndrome in the family
- √ Syncope with abnormal cardiac exam
- √ Syncope with abnormal EKG

DIFFERENTIAL DIAGNOSIS OF SYNCOPE

Cardiac

- Vasovagal syncope
- Orthostatic hypotension
- Heart block
- Arrhythmias (unprovoked or exercise induced)
- Carotid sinus disease *(Abrupt neck movement)*
- Myocarditis
- Cardiomyopathy
- Orthostatic hypotension
- coronary artery anomaly
- Atrial myxoma

Neurologic

- AVM
- Migraines
- Elevated ICP
- Head trauma
- Seizures
- Stroke, TIA

Situational

- Syncope with coughing, micturition, defecation, straining

Pulmonary

- Severe Pulmonary hypertension

Other

- Dehydration
- breath-holding spells in children
- Hyperventilation
- Dysautonomia
- adrenal insufficiency
- Hypoglycemia
- Psychogenic (Pseudo syncope)

PALPITATION

Onset
Lasts for
Regular or irregular rhythm
Frequency
Lasts for...
At Rest?
Aggravating
Alleviating
Associated
- Chest pain
- SOB
- Sweating/ Jitteriness
- Nausea/ vomiting
- Hand tremors
- Recent Wt loss
- Diarrhea
- Polyurea
- Anxiety/ Agitation
- Neurological deficits

FOR INFANTS:
Feeding difficulty, Tiredness, Rapid breathing, Cyanosis, Sweating with feeding

PMH: cardiac dz, thyroid problems

Medication: caffeine/ stimulants
Drugs causing prolonged QT interval
Other meds

FH: FH of similar sxs, cardiac disease run in the family, sudden death or FH of Prolonged QT syndrome,

Social Hx: smoking, illicit drug abuse

PERTIENT PHYSICAL EXAM

Check vitals HR, BP, O2 saturation

GEN: signs of distress, hydration status, perfusion

FUNDSCOPY: papilledema

NECK: thyroidomegaly

CHEST: breath sounds, wheeze, crackles

CVS: Precordial thrill, Heart sounds, murmur, gallop, rub

Carotid bruits, peripheral pulses

ABD: hepatomegaly

DIFFERENTIAL DIAGNOSIS

Sinus tachycardia

- Fever, sepsis
- Dehydration
- Anemia
- Hyperthyroidism
- Hypoglycemia
- Stimulant overdose
- Anxiety/ Panic attack

Non-sinus tachycardia *(underlying cardiac disease)*

- Arrythmias: SVT, AF, A feb, ...
- WBW syndrome
- Sick sinus syndrome

EDEMA

Onset
Extension Localized /Generalized
Previous Episodes
Course: worsening, Constant
If Generalized:

- Where 1st started
- Progress pattern
- Change with daytime

If Localized:

- Location
- Painful/ painless
- Insect bite
- Hx of trauma

Aggravating factors
Relieving factors
Recent URI
Decrease urine output
Associated Sxs

- Fever
- Wt or appetite loss
- Hard time putting shoes on (if LL)
- Abdominal distension
- Nausea/ vomiting
- Difficulty breathing
- Vomiting
- Skin rash or itchiness

PMH: Chronic diarrhea, Heart or renal disease
PSH: any previous surgeries

Meds:

Allergies:

Family Hx:

Social Hx:

PERTIENT PHYSICAL EXAM

Check vitals, O2 saturation
GEN: signs of distress, perfusion, pitting /non-pitting edema?
EYE: periorbital edema, papilledema
CHEST: breath sounds, wheeze, crackles, dullness on percussion
CVS: Heart sounds, murmur, gallop, rub, peripheral pulses, LL edema, peripheral pulses
ABD/GENITALIAL: Abdominal distension, shifting dullness, organomegaly, sacral/ genital edema
SKIN: erythema, tenderness

DIFFERENTIAL DIAGNOSIS

Generalized edema

- Congestive heart failure
- Renal failure
- Hepatic failure
- Protein losing enteropathy, kwashiorkor *(in children)*
- Allergic reaction/ anaphylaxis
- Lymphatic / thoracic duct obstruction
- Nephrotic syndrome
- Venous return obstruction
- Iatrogenic fluid overload
- Sodium retention, hypothyroidism
- Pregnancy
- Medication side effects *(CCB, steroids)*

Localized edema

- Trauma
- Infection (cellulitis)
- Allergy
- Insect bite
- Localized lymphatic obstruction

COUGH

Duration
Character
Dry/Productive
- Amount of sputum
- Color of sputum
- Blood
- Odor

Diurnal variation:
- Diurnal cough *(habit, psychogenic)*
- Night cough *(sinusitis, asthma*

Exposure to Sick person/ TB
Aggravating factors
Alleviating factors
Treatments used
Odor
Recent URI
Associated sxs:
- Fever
- Nasal congestion
- Night sweats
- Wt loss
- Loss of appetite
- SOB
- Chest pain

PMH:

PSH: Any previous surgery, when, indication, complications

Meds Hx: ACEI, other medications

FH:

Social Hx: smoking, recent travel, pets, Animal exposure

PERTIENT PHYSICAL EXAM

Check vitals and O2 saturation

GEN: Ill/ toxic appearing, Built (Obesity, malnourished, cachexic)
NOSE/THROAT: *(atopy → pale swollen nasal mucosa and cobblestone in back of throat, eczema)*
CHEST: Grunting, retractions suprasternal, intercostal, subcostal retractions, decrease air entry, wheezing or crackles **(***FB aspiration localized decrease air entry and wheeze)*
CVS: murmur or gallop, poor pulses
Peripheral edema *(renal or cardiac cause)*
ABD: Severe
Abdominal
distension or ascites
*(compression on
lung)*

DIFFERENTIAL DIAGNOSIS

- URI
- Allergic rhinitis
- Sinusitis
- Asthma
- Pneumonia
- Bronchitis/ bronchiectasis
- Pleuritis
- Cystic fibrosis
- Primary ciliary dyskinesia
- Pulmonary TB
- COPD
- GERD / Chronic reflux
- Foreign body
- Ciliary dyskinesia syndromes
- Smoking

SHORTNESS OF BREATH

Duration
Onset sudden / gradual
Course: intermittent / constant
Severity SOB at rest or on exertion
Aggravated by
- Exercise, position, Anxiety
- Exposures *(medications/sting /dust)*

Relieved by
- Rest, sitting up
- Inhaler use *(Dose/ how frequent/ last used)*

Associated sxs:
- Fever
- Cough / Nocturnal cough
- Rhinorrhea, Nasal congestion
- Chest Pain/Tightness
- Wheeze
- Cyanosis
- Wt or appetite Loss
- Night sweats
- Lip / Facial swelling
- hives/ itchiness
- Rash
- Joint pain or swelling

PMH:
Recurrent respiratory infections, Hx of cardiac problems, Hx Asthma *(frequency using rescue bronchodilators, last ED visit, Hx of ICU admission or intubation)*
Hx of atopy (eczema, allergic rhinitis, urticaria)
Hx of neurological weakness, or swallowing problems *(aspiration)*
Meds: for Inhaler use, rescue or controller (Dose/ how frequent/Compliance)

Allergies:
FH: Atopy (asthma, eczema, allergic rhinitis) in family
Social Hx:
Smoking/ passive smoking, pets at home
Recent travel, Hx of TB contact

PERTIENT PHYSICAL EXAM

ASK Pt to COUNT to 10 (if applicable)
Check vitals and O2 saturation
GEN: Ill/ toxic appearing, built *(Obesity, malnourished, cachexic)*, sings of acute distress
ENT: pale swollen nasal mucosa and cobblestone in back of throat
SKIN: eczema
CHEST: grunting, retractions suprasternal, intercostal, subcostal retractions, decrease air entry, wheezing or crackles *(FB aspiration localized decrease air entry and wheeze)*
CVS: murmur or gallop, poor pulses
Peripheral edema *(renal or cardiac cause)*
ABD: Severe Abdominal distension or ascites *(compression on lung)*

DIFFERENTIAL DIAGNOSIS

Pulmonary

- Pneumonia
- Pulmonary TB
- Asthma exacerbation
- COPD exacerbation
- Spontaneous pneumothorax
- Pulmonary embolism

Cardiac

- MI
- Pleuritis
- Cardiac tamponed

Miscellaneous

- Anaphylaxis
- Malignancy
- Neuromuscular diseases
- Sarcoidosis

STRIDOR

Duration
Inspiratory or expiratory
Onset: sudden, gradual
Course: worsening, constant
Frequency: intermittent, Static
Severity: at rest (sever) or only with activity/crying
Change with position
Aggravating factors
Relieving factors
Associated Sxs

- Cyanosis
- Difficulty breathing
- Cough
- Fever
- Drooling
- Foreign body aspiration
- Hx of trauma
- Preceding URI symptoms
- Rash / hives/ facial or lip swelling

PMH:

- Hx of prematurity in children
- Hx of intubation
- Hx of anaphylaxis
- Hx of neck masses

PSH:

- Neck surgery
- Cardiac surgery
- PDA ligation

Meds Hx:

Allergy: hx of food, medications allergy

Family Hx: Hx of anaphylaxis
Social Hx: Active or passive smoking

PERTIENT PHYSICAL EXAM

Check vital signs and O2 saturation

GEN: toxic / non-toxic appearing, dysmorphic features, drooling, agitation, cyanosis

DO NOT EXAMINE THE THROAT

LUNGS: Inspiratory or expiratory stridor, retractions suprasternal, intercostal, subcostal retractions, decrease air entry, wheezing or crackles
CVS: *murmur or gallop, poor pulses*
Peripheral edema (*renal or cardiac cause*)

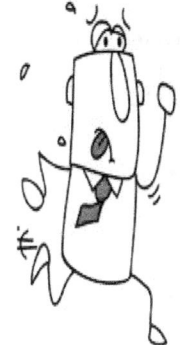

STRIDOR CAN BE...

Inspiratory → Upper airway (extrathoracic)

Expiratory → lower airway (intrathoracic)

Biphasic indicates severe stridor

DIFFERENTIAL DIAGNOSIS

- Epiglottitis
- Croup (laryngotracheobronchitis)
- Laryngitis
- Tracheitis
- Hypocalcemia
- Laryngospasm
- Subglottic stenosis
- Foreign body aspiration
- Anaphylactic reaction
- Laryngomalacia/ tracheomalacia
- Subglottic web / hemangioma

Extrinsic compression from:

- Vascular
- Branchial/thyroglossal cyst
- Cystic hygroma
- Tumor (laryngeal, mediastinal)
- Goiter or thyroid masses

HEMAPTYSIS

Duration:
Amount: streaks, clots, .. tbs/cup
Mixed with sputum or not
Color: bright red, brown, coffee ground
Course: worsening, constant
Frequency: intermittent, static
Previous episodes
Hx of Trauma
Associated Sxs

- Cough
- Fever
- SOB
- Chest pain
- Wt or appetite loss
- Night sweating
- Hoarseness of voice
- Skin rash
- Painful calf swelling (DVT)
- Bleeding from other body sites

PMH: hx bleeding disorders or vasculitis, Hx of TB, renal disease

PSH: Recent bronchoscopy or lung surgery

Meds Hx:
Anticoagulants, Immunosuppressive therapy

Vaccination Hx:

Allergy:

Family Hx: bleeding disorders, malignancy, TB exposure

Social Hx:
Smoking
IV drug abuse
Recent travel
Occupation *(exposures, e.g. asbestos)*

PERTIENT PHYSICAL EXAM

Check vitals and O2 saturation

GEN: Ill/ toxic appearing, pale, cyanosis, cachexic
NOSE: nasal bleeding or perforation
CHEST: retractions suprasternal, intercostal, subcostal retractions, decrease air entry, wheezing or crackles, friction rub
CVS: murmur or gallop, pulses
Abd: hepatosplenomegaly or ascites
Ext: clubbing, cyanosis
Skin: petechiae, bruises, ecchymosis

DIFFERENTIAL DIAGNOSIS

- Bronchitis
- Bronchiectasis
- Lung tumor
- Pulmonary TB
- Lung fungal infection
- Lung abscess
- Pneumonia
- Vasculitis (*Wegner/ Goodpasture synd.*)
- Pulmonary embolism or lung infarction
- Iatrogenic during bronchoscope
- Trauma

VOMITING

Onset sudden/ gradual
Duration
Number of episodes
Projectile/ forceful/ forceless
Amount
Content
Color: bilious or non-bilious
Any blood with vomit
Timing

- Early morning
- Soon after eating
- Later > 1hr of mealtime

Last bowel movement *(think of intestinal obstruction)*
Associated sxs

- Fever
- Nausea
- Dysphagia
- Regurgitation
- Diarrhea
- Abdominal pain
- Abdominal distension
- Headache
- Neck stiffness/ photophobia
- Chest pain / diaphoresis
- Jaundice
- Dysuria/ hematuria
- Wt loss, night sweats

Last menstrual period in females *(pregnancy)*
Possible ingestion of foreign body
Any toxic or recent new ingestions
Hx of abdominal trauma

PMH: Hx of DM, kidney disease. Migraine. Peptic ulcer disease, reflux, any other chronic disease
Hx of use of macrolides in newborn

PSH: any previous surgery

Meds Hx:
Any medications including
Vitamins or supplements

Allergy:

Family Hx: Any family member with similar sxs
FH of migraine or cyclic vomiting syndrome

Social Hx:
Diet
Recent travel
Heavy marijuana use
Illicit drug abuse

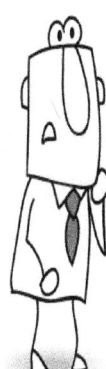

RED FLAGS FOR EMESIS

- Bilious emesis
- Dehydration
- Signs of shock
- hematemesis (especially with the first episode)
- Abdominal distension and absent bowel sounds
- Early morning or wakes a patient from sleep

DDx of projectile emesis in infants

- Pyloric stenosis
- Antral web

PERTIENT PHYSICAL EXAM

Check Vital signs

GEN: Signs of dehydration, Parotid enlargement

FUNDOSCOPY: papilledema

ABD: abdominal distension, tenderness, visible bowel loop, bowel sounds

Pelvic tenderness and pelvic exam

SKIN: jaundice, orange tinted skin *(hypervitaminosis A)*

NEURO: Tense AF (in toddlers) nystagmus, weakness or abnormal reflexes

DIFFERENTIAL DIAGNOSIS

Acute emesis

- Small bowel obstruction, SMA syndrome
- Intussusception
- Volvulus
- Appendicitis
- Foreign body or drug ingestion,
- Incarcerated hernia
- Intestinal adhesions
- GERD/ Peptic ulcer disease
- Pancreatitis
- Cholelithiasis
- Choledocholithiasis
- UTI
- Obstructive uropathy
- Ovarian torsion
- Pregnancy
- Elevated ICP
- CNS infection
- Head injury
- Inborn errors of metabolism
- Adrenal insufficiency
- Eating disorders
- Food allergy
- Anaphylaxis
- Porphyria
- Hypervitaminosis
- Chemotherapy

chronic emesis

- Cyclic vomiting
- Rumination

HEMATEMESIS

Duration
Previous Episodes
Course: worsening, static
Color bright red, brown, coffee ground
Amount
Number of episodes
Blood present with first emesis?
Blood present with each emesis?
Hx of trauma/ FB ingestion
Associated Sxs

- Prior persistent non-bloody emesis
- Abdominal pain
- Dysphagia
- Dyspepsia
- Bloody stool/ black stool
- Chest pain
- Wt loss/ night sweats

PMH:
Hx of GERD or peptic ulcer
Hx of Esophageal varies
Hx of Hepatic failure/ Cirrhosis
Hx of bleeding disorders

PSH: any previous surgeries

Meds Hx:
Anticoagulants, ASA or other NSAID use

Allergy:

Family Hx:
FH of bleeding disorders

Social Hx:
Smoking
Alcohol or illicit drugs abuse
Recent travel

PERTIENT PHYSICAL EXAM

Check vital signs

GEN: Pallor, signs of dehydration

SKIN: bruises, petechiae, icterus, palmer erythema, spider Navi

ABD: abdominal distension, tenderness, organomegaly, masses, shifting dullness, bowel sounds

DIFFERENTIAL DIAGNOSIS

- Bleeding peptic ulcer
- Mallory Weiss syndrome
- Swallowed blood (from nose or lung)
- Bleeding esophageal varices
- Gastric erosions
- Esophageal carcinoma
- Gastric carcinoma
- Traumatic injury from ingested FB
- Ingestion of corrosives
- Angiodysplasia/ AVM
- Bleeding disorders

DYSPHAGIA

Duration
Onset: sudden, gradual
Difficulty swallowing fluid, solid or both
Progression: worsening, constant
Painful or Painless
Intermittent or constant (*intermittent in esophageal spasms*)
Level: neck, upper or mid chest
Difficulty initiating swallowing
Aggravating factors
Alleviating factors
Associated Sxs

- Chocking
- Regurgitation
- Drooling
- Night cough (aspirations)
- Halitosis
- Chest pain
- Neck swelling
- Wt / Appetite loss

Possible FB ingestion
Do you take meds with water? or do you take your bills immediately before going to bed? *(pill esophagitis)*
PMH:
Hx of reflux, GERD
Hx of radiation exposure
Hx of asthma or atopy and food allergy
Stroke or neurological disorders

PSH: any previous surgeries

Meds Hx:

Allergy: Hx of food allergy

Family Hx: Hx of dysphagia in the family
FH of autoimmune diseases
Social Hx:
Recent travel, Occupation
Smoking and Illicit drug abuse

PERTIENT PHYSICAL EXAM

Check vital signs

GEN: pallor, malnourished

NECK: mass, swelling, lymphadenopathy

SKIN: scleroderma

LUNG: crackles (*due to aspiration*)

ABD: abdominal distension, organomegaly, masses

DIFFERENTIAL DIAGNOSIS

Intrinsic Mechanical obstruction
- Stricture
- Pharyngeal mass
- Esophageal mass

Extrinsic Mechanical obstruction
- Retrosternal thyroid
- Right side aorta
- Aortic aneurysm
- Lung mass
- Mediastinal mass

Motility disorders
- Achalasia
- MS
- Bulbar palsy
- Myasthenia gravis
- Esophageal spasm
- Scleroderma

Others
- Esophagitis

JAUNDICE

Duration:
Onset: sudden, gradual
Course: worsening, constant
Previous episodes
Any toxic ingestion including wild mushroom
Associated Sxs

- Fever
- Fatigue/ night sweats
- Wt loss
- Pruritis
- Nausea and vomiting
- Abdominal pain
- Abdominal distension
- Dark urine
- Pale stool or steatorrhea
- Bruising
- Hematuria
- Joint pain
- Rash
- Neurological deficits like dysarthria, dystonia, ataxia, dementia or behavioral changes *(young adult, think of Wilson's dz.)*

LMP *(in females)*

PMH:

Hx of blood transfusion
PSH: any previous surgeries

Meds Hx:
Acetaminophen intake *(calculate daily dose)*
Any supplements or herbal medications

Family Hx: Hx of jaundice, hepatic or hemolytic disorders

Social Hx:
Recent travel
Alcohol intake
IV drug abuse

PERTIENT PHYSICAL EXAM

Check vital signs

GEN: ill/toxic appearing, malnourished, asterixis *(flapping tremors)*
EYE: icteric sclera, Kayser-Fisher ring, cataract
SKIN: icterus, spider angiomas, palmer erythema, excoriation marks, bronze hyperpigmentation, petechiae, bruises
CHEST: gynecomastia *(in males)*
ABD: abdominal distension, hepatosplenomegaly, liver span & texture, shifting dullness or fluid thrill
NEURO: lethargy, mini-mental status *(encephalopathy)*, neurological deficits

DIFFERENTIAL DIAGNOSIS

Age of patient is very important for DDx

- Gallstone disease
- Infectious hepatitis, HAV, HBV, HCV, EBV, CMV ….
- Acute hemolysis (sickle cell, G6PD deficiency)
- Pregnancy, HELP syndrome
- Hemoglobinuria
- Non- Alcoholic Fatty Liver disease (NAFLD)
- Alcoholic cirrhosis
- Gilbert syndrome
- Alagille syndrome
- Criglar- Najjar syndrome
- Dubin- Johnson syndrome
- Rotor Syndrome
- Wilson's disease
- Hemochromatosis
- Primary biliary cirrhosis
- Primary sclerosing cholangitis
- Pancreatic carcinoma
- Biliary carcinoma

NEONATAL JAUNDICE

Ethnicity *(Asians are high risk population)*
Duration
Onset: 1st day of life or later
Course: progressing/ regressing
Color of stool & Urine
# of wet diapers in last 24hr
Birth wt & % of wt loss
Maternal & baby Blood groups
Associated Sxs

- Fever
- Lethargy/ Fussiness
- Feeding intolerance
- Seizures
- Rash

Prenatal Hx
Maternal diseases GDM, pre-eclampsia..
Hx of maternal infections *(rash or fever)* during pregnancy
(Review maternal labs if possible)
Maternal medications

Birth Hx:
Gestational age
Birth wt
Mode of delivery *(birth trauma)*
Delayed cord clamp
Newborn screen result

Meds Hx: current medication, any herbal remedies

Family Hx:
Parental consanguinity
Previous siblings with neonatal jaundice
family members with jaundice
FH of hemolytic disorders
FH of Splenectomy

PERTIENT PHYSICAL EXAM

Check vital signs and Wt, Ht, HC
GEN: ill-appearing, lethargy, dysmorphic features, pallor
EYES: icteric sclera, cataract *(check red reflex)*
HEAD: microcephaly, Cephalohematoma
SKIN extension of jaundice, bruises, petechiae, rash, scratch marks
CVS: murmur *(TORCH, Alagille syndrome)*
ABD: distended, hepatomegaly, splenomegaly, RUQ mass *(choledochal cyst)*
NEURO: lethargy, hypo/hypertonia, seizures

DIFFERENTIAL DIAGNOSIS

Unconjugated hyperbilirubinemia

- Physiological
- ABO/ Rh incompatibility
- Breast feeding (dehydration)
- Breast milk jaundice
- Hemolytic disorders, such as G6PD def, pyruvate kinase def., spherocytosis, thalassemia,
- RBCs breakdown from hematomas, hemorrhages or polycythemia
- Medications side effects
- DIC

Conjugated hyperbilirubinemia

- Biliary atresia
- Sepsis/ TORCH infection
- Neonatal hepatitis (infectious or idiopathic)
- Hypothyroidism
- Galactosemia or other inborn errors of metabolism
- Hemolytic disorders, DIC
- Choledochal cyst

DIARRHEA

Duration:
Onset: sudden, gradual
Course: worsening, constant
Number of episodes
Amount
Stool color
Blood or mucous with stool
Tenesmus (*sense of incomplete emptying*)
Difficulty flashing stool
Relation to food (Wheat/ dairy products)
Any recent change in diet
Aggravating factors
Relieving factors
Associated Sxs

- Fever
- Nausea or Vomiting
- Abdominal pain
- Abdominal bloating
- Wt loss, night sweating
- Arthritis
- Conjunctivitis
- Hot flashing
- Heat intolerance

PMH:
Any chronic illness, recent hospitalization, Hx of chronic constipation (*overflow diarrhea*)

PSH:
Meds Hx:

- Laxative use
- Recent antibiotic use
- Supplements or herbal medications

Vaccination Hx:

Allergy:

Family Hx:
Any family member with similar sxs
Inflammatory bowel disease. Irritable bowel disease, malignancy

Social Hx:

Attending daycare if children, working in daycare, Any pets, recent travel

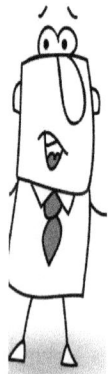

> Normal stool frequency in breastfed infant: once every 7 days or 7 times a day

CAUSES OF BLOODY DIARRHEA

- Infectious
- Shigella dysenteries
- Campylobacter enteritis
- Enteroinvasive E Coli
- Enterohemorrhagic E Coli
- Entamoeba Histolytica
- Croh's disease
- Ulcerative Colitis
- Diverticulitis
- Colonic Carcinoma

PERTIENT PHYSICAL EXAM

Vital sings & parametric measurements

GEN: sings of dehydration, built

MOUTH: oral ulcers, dry lips & mucous membranes

CVS: HR, perfusion, pulses (*hydration status*)

ABD: abdominal distension, tenderness, masses, bowel sounds

MSK: clubbing, arthritis

DIFFERENTIAL DIAGNOSIS

Acute Diarrhea

- Infectious (viral, bacterial, parasites)
- Lactose intolerance
- Medications (laxative, certain antibiotics)
- Overflow diarrhea

Chronic diarrhea

- Cystic fibrosis
- Celiac disease
- Short bowel syndrome
- Pancreatic insufficiency
- Post-infectious enteropathy
- Malabsorption syndromes
- Inflammatory bowel disease
- Irritable bowel disease
- Secretory tumors (VIPoma, Carcinoid tumor, gastrinoma)
- Hyperthyroidism
- Immune deficiency syndromes

CONSTIPATION

Duration *(when was last bowel movement?)*

Frequency of BM
What is normal stool frequency
Stool Consistency *(Bristol chart)*
What is normal consistency of stool
Color of stool
Any bloody stool (mixed/ outside)
Any pain with defecation
Interventions done (enema, laxative, suppository ...)
Associated Sxs

- Fever
- Nausea/ vomiting
- Loss of appetite
- Weight loss/ gain
- Abdominal Pain
- Abdominal distension
- Fatigue
- Cold intolerance
- Dysuria
- Alternating diarrhea & constipation with bloating

PMH:
FOR CHILDREN: (Hx of chronic constipation / since when?
Did pass meconium on first 48 hr of life?
Newborn screen negative for CF or thyroid problems)
Hx of hypothyroidism
Any chronic illness

PSH: Previous abdominal surgery or radiation

Meds Hx: Laxative use, Calcium / Iron supplements, Opiate, others

Family Hx: FH of thyroid disorders, malignancy or colonic polyps

Social Hx: Diet/ fiber intake/ fluid intake
Exercise, Opiate abuse

PERTIENT PHYSICAL EXAM

GEN: built, flat affect, pallor

NECK: Thyroid, lymph nodes

ABD: bowel sounds, abdominal distension, abdominal mass, organomegaly

PR: fissure, perianal soiling, skin tag, perianal rash, anal sphincter tone, stool in rectum or blood, anal wink

NEURO: decrease lower extremities reflexes & tone

BACK: sacral dimple, lipoma, tuft of hair

DIFFERENTIAL DIAGNOSIS

Functional constipation in children (*Dx of exclusion*)

Psychosocial

- low fiber diet and sedentary life
- Depression
- Irritable bowel syndrome

Metabolic/ Endocrine

- Hypothyroidism
- Hyperparathyroidism
- Diabetes
- Hypercalcemia
- Hypomagnesaemia
- Hypokalemia
- Uremia
- Lead poisoning

Obstruction

- Anal fissure
- Fecal impaction
- Stricture
- Volvulus
- Colonic polyp

Infections

- Botulism
- Chagas disease
- Tetanus
- Diverticulitis

Neurogenic disorders

- Hirschsprung disease
- Autonomic neuropathy
- Spinal cord compression by neoplasm
- Spinal cord injury
- Tethered spinal cord
- MS

Medications side effect

- Anticholinergic
- Antidepressant
- Calcium supplements
- Iron supplements
- Antispasmodics
- Cholestyramine
- Verapamil

PEDIATRIC FAILURE TO THRIVE

Duration/ When noticed?
How is appetite?
Nutritional History:

- caloric intake (recall last 24-hour diet)
- Food type (formula/table food)
- **For breast fed** *(How is mother's milk supply, if mother pumps milk, how much she gets?* how long baby spend on each breast?)
- **For formula fed**: (Formula's name, Amount oz, how many calories per oz? formula preparation)
- Feeding Frequency *(Is feeding is scheduled or on demand?)*
- Time to finish feeds
- **For children eating table food** (Meal size, Frequency, Any dietary restrictions)
- Access to formula/food

Feeding problems
- Poor sucking
- Fatigue or sweating during feeding
- Spit up/ vomiting

Associated Sxs

- Fever, chills, appetite changes, night sweats
- Fussiness/ Lethargy
- Diarrhea/ constipation
- Color of stool
- Bloody stools
- Abdominal distension
- SOB/ wheezing
- Rashes

Perinatal Hx:

- maternal diseases or infections, smoking, drug abuse, Hx of prematurity IUGR or SGA.
- birth Wt, gestational age, congenital anomalies
- postnatal complications

PMH: recurrent infections, previous hospitalization, chronic illnesses

PSH: any previous surgeries

Meds Hx: any current medications

Vaccination Hx:

Allergy:

Family Hx: previous sudden infant death, any diseases run in the family

Social Hx:
Parents education and financial situation
Parental smoking or drug abuse
Parental depression

PERTINENT PHYSICAL EXAM	DIFFERENTIAL DIAGNOSIS

Review medical records for previous Wt, and growth charts and calculate daily/ weekly wt gain (if possible)

Observe parent-child interaction

Parametric measures (Centiles) / Vitals / O2 saturation

GEN: Built (malnourished/ cachexia/ muscle wasting) dehydration, ill appearance, dysmorphic or developmental delay

HEAD: head size, signs of trauma, temporal wasting
LYMPH NODES: Cervical or supraclavicular lymphadenopathy.
EYES: sunken eyes, cataracts icterus,

MOUTH: Cheilosis, glossitis, teeth erosions, oropharyngeal lesions
NECK: Thyromegaly, LAD

SKIN: Pallor, jaundice, rash, bruises or signs of trauma

CHEST: Barrel shaped chest, rhonchi.
Heart: Displaced point of maximal impulse, murmur, gallop, peripheral edema
Abdomen: abdominal distension, organomegaly or masses

Neuro: Tone, power, reflexes, sensation, CN II-XII. Gait

Genitalia: Hypospadias (obstructive uropathy)

Inadequate caloric intake

- Inadequate caloric intake (unintentional)
- Poor breast milk supply,
- Poor feeding techniques due to tongue tie, cleft lip or palate, new or single parent
- Severe gastroesophageal reflux
- Diluted formula
- Neglect/ abuse

Inadequate nutrient absorption

- celiac disease
- Cystic fibrosis
- Milk protein allergy
- Inborn errors of metabolism
- Biliary atresia
- Malabsorption syndromes

Increase metabolic demands

- Congenital heart disease
- Chronic lung disease
- Recurrent infections
- Hyperthyroidism
- Malignancy
- Renal failure

ABDOMINAL PAIN

Location
Duration
Onset: sudden, gradual
Character: colicky, stabbing, dull, tearing, ….
Severity
Course: worsening, constant
Frequency intermittent, static
If intermittent: how frequent & lasts for..
Radiation
Aggravating factors
Relieving factors
Previous episodes
Hx of Trauma
Associated Sxs

- Fever
- Nausea/ vomiting *(ask Duration/ Frequency & ABC amount, blood, color)*
- Diarrhea
- Constipation
- Bloody stool
- Appetite/ Wt loss
- Night sweats
- Painful urination
- Hematuria
- Sore throat

Females with abdominal pain:
Menstrual Hx, Vaginal bleeding or discharge, sexual Hx
Males with abdominal pain:
Testicular pain or swelling, penile discharge, sexual Hx

PMH: any chronic diseases
PSH: previous abdominal or pelvic surgeries

Meds Hx: current medications

Family Hx: similar sxs in the family, FH of oral ulcers, IBD, irritable bowel syndrome

Social Hx: Recent travel

PERTIENT PHYSICAL EXAM

Perform complete physical exam with focus on detailed abdominal exam

ABDOMINAL EXAM
Inspect: distension, scars *(location, healing stages)*, dilated veins, visible pulsation, bruising, hernias (ask pt to cough) drains or stomas.
Palpate: all for quadrants
Superficially to look for guarding, tenderness (location) CVA tenderness or rebound tenderness. Deeply to look for organomegaly or masses, or to perform specific signs *(see below)*
Percuss: to measure liver span or to look for shifting dullness.
Auscultate: bowel sounds or bruits

Positive Sings of appendicitis:
performing these maneuvers can worsen RLQ pain

- **Mc Burney point tenderness**
- **Rebound tenderness**
- **Heel tap or jumping up and down**
- **Dunphy's sing** (pain on coughing)
- **Rovsing's sign** (LLQ palpation)
- **Psoas sing** (raising R leg)
- **Obturator signs** (internal rotation of R hip with flexed R knee)

DIFFERENTIAL DIAGNOSIS

DDx depends on the sites of pain *(which quadrant?)*, chronicity, associated sxs and patient's age

Abdominal Pain Red flags

- Awaken from sleep
- Localized pain
- Fever
- Wt loss
- Bloody stool
- Rash
- Joint pain
- MM ulcers
- FH of documented ulcers or FH of IBD

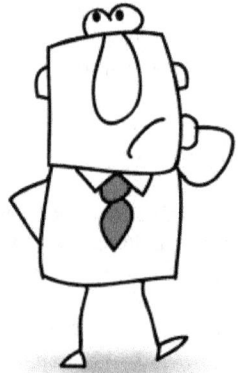

BLOODY STOOL/ BLEEDING PER RECTUM

Duration
Color of blood: bright red, dark red, or black tarry sticky stool?

Is it with every bowel movement?
Is it mixed with stool, separate from stool or when wiping?
Amount: strikes, clots, ….
Stool consistency
Any recent changes in bowel movement?
Bleeding from other body parts
Associated sxs:
- Abdominal pain
- Nausea/ vomiting
- Diarrhea/ constipation
- Painful defecation
- Palpitation
- Dizziness or syncope
- Fatigue
- Wt or appetite loss
- Night sweats

For infants with bloody stool
Feeding Hx, type of formula or breast milk
Associated fussiness, vomiting, abdominal distension, stool caliber & consistency

PMH: constipation, IBD, autoimmune diseases

Meds Hx: current meds, anticoagulants, NSAID

Allergies:

FH: colon cancer or familial colonic polyps

Social Hx:
diet (low fiber), smoking, alcohol or drugs abuse, Recent travel

TREMORS

Duration:
Unilateral or bilateral
At rest or with movement
Onset: sudden, gradual
Course: worsening, Constant
Frequency intermittent, Static
Character – rapid or slow
Aggravating factors (e.g. stress, fatigue)
Relieving factors *(e.g. alcohol)*
Caffeine intake
Associated Sxs

- Abnormal gait
- Frequent falls/ Imbalance
- Rigidity
- Limb weakness/numbness
- Speech difficulty
- dementia or Confusion
- Hallucination
- Wt loss
- Palpitation
- Heat intolerance
- Neck mass
- Anxiety episodes

PMH:
Hx of thyroid disease, seizure disorders, asthma or COPD, DM

PSH: any previous episodes

Meds Hx: B agonist use, Stimulants, Thyroxine, Insulins/ oral antidiabetics
Others

Family Hx: FH of tremors, Parkinson's disease

Social Hx
Illicit drug or alcohol abuse
Occupation/ exposures to Heavy metal, pesticides, cyanide, arsenic, CO

PERTINENT PHYSICAL EXAM

Check vital signs

GEN: anxious, flat affect, low BMI, observe tremors at rest or on movement

SKIN: palmer erythema, spider Navi, warm sweaty skin

NECK: Thyroid exam

EYE: exophthalmos, lid lag, Kayser-Fleischer ring

CVS: Tachycardia, irregular rhythm

ABD: Hepatomegaly, shifting dullness

NEURO: Tone, reflexes, cranial nerves, coordination, Romberg test, and gait

Cerebellar sings: dysdiadochokinesia (*impaired rapid, alternating hand movements*), ataxia, nystagmus, intention tremor, scanning dysarthria, heel–shin test positive

DIFFERENTIAL DIAGNOSIS

Fine Tremors

- Essential tremors
- Hyperthyroidism
- Fatigue
- Anxiety
- Acute drug/alcohol withdrawal
- Hypoglycemia
- Medications side effect
    - Excess caffeine
    - Sympathomimetics
    - SSRI
    - Lithium
    - Levothyroxine

Coarse Tremors

- Parkinsonian syndromes
- Cerebellar dysfunction
- Wilson's disease
- CO_2 retention
- Hepatic Failure

Causes of unilateral tremors

- Parkinsonism
- Unilateral cerebellar lesions

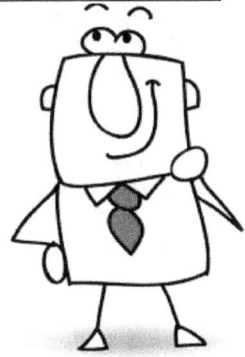

DM FOLLOW UP

Is it type 1 or 2
When was diagnosed?
Who diagnosed you?
Initial presenting sxs
Last follow up
Last HbA1c
Home monitoring?
Any recent DKA
What medication taking
Medication compliance
Any new medication changes
Medication side effects
Is your blood sugar controlled?
Any new symptoms
- Vomiting
- Abdominal pain
- Blurry vision
- Weakness/ numbness
- TIA
- Foot ulcers or injury
- Erectile dysfunction

PMH: *(Cardiovascular disease risk factors)*
- Hypertension
- hypercholesterolemia
- Previous stroke/TIA
- MI

Hx of Recurrent infections

Compliance with annual check up
- Last eye exam
- Last urine microalbumin & renal function
- Last lipid panel
- Thyroid function test *(if at risk e.g. Down syndrome and Celiac dz)*

Immunization Hx: includes annual flu vaccine and Pneumococcal *(according to patient age)*

DYSURIA/ PAINFUL URINATION

Duration
Frequency
Urgency
Urine stream changes
Hematuria
Use of bubble bath *(changes PH for urethral flora)*
Holding behaviors
Hx of Indwelling catheter
Associated sxs

- Fever
- Chills/ Rigors
- Nausea/ Vomiting
- Abdominal pain *(ask SOCRATES)*
- Diarrhea
- Vag/penile discharge
- Genital itchiness
- Genital rash

PMH: hx of recurrent UTI, Chronic constipation, Urinary tract abnormalities, DM, or any other chronic diseases

PSH: Any abdominal or urological surgery

Meds Hx: Current use of any medications

Family Hx: Renal diseases

Social Hx:

Detailed sexual hx *(see page 88)*

DIFFERENTIAL DIAGNOSIS

- UTI
- Pyelonephritis
- STI
- Urolithiasis

HEMATOURIA

Duration:
How did you know it was blood?
Color? Bright red / brown cola
Number of episodes
Hx of Previous episodes
Frequency: intermittent, static with each void
Diurnal variation
Course: worsening or static
Amount/ Presence of clot
Relation to urine stream

- Beginning (*Urethra/prostate*)
- Mid (*Bladder*)
- End (*Kidney*)

Urine stream changes: Dripping...weak...
Sensation of incomplete voiding or straining
Bleeding from other body sites
Hx of trauma to genital area
Hx of vigorous exercise
Diet (*beetroot turns urine red*)
Associated sxs

- Fever
- Burning with voiding (UTI)
- Frequency
- Urgency
- Flank pain or CVA pain
- Facial swelling
- Lower limb edema
- rash, arthritis, lung disease (rheumatological diseases)
- Epistaxis / Hemoptysis (Wegner syndromes/Good Postures Syndrome)

Hx of Concurrent or recent URI or skin infection

Menstrual Hx in females *(see page 88)*

PMH: Renal stones, Bleeding disorders, Recurrent Urinary tract infections, Cancer

PSH: Any previous urinary tract surgery

Medications Rifampicin/nitrofurantoin (turn *urine red*)
Anticoagulants/antiplatelets
Vaccination history
Allergies:
Family Hx:
FH of renal stones,
renal diseases, family member on dialysis
FH of deafness or using hearing aid (Alport syndrome)
FH of bleeding disorders
Social Hx: Smoking, recent travel, occupation

DIFFERENTIAL DIAGNOSIS

Non-glomerular gross hematuria
- UTI
- Stone
- Hypercalciuria
- PCKD
- Renal trauma
- Papillary necrosis
- Interstitial nephritis
- Hemorrhagic cystitis
- Urethrorrhagia (*terminal hamartia in adolescent, self-resolved*)
- Sickle cell trait or disease
- Renal Vein thrombosis
- Schistosoma Haematobium
- Renal/ bladder/ prostate carcinoma

Glomerular causes of gross hematuria
- IgA nephropathy
- Post-infectious glomerulonephritis
- Alport syndrome
- Vasculitis e.g. Wegner Granulomatosis
- Thin basement membrane disease (familial)

ENURESIS IN CHILDREN

Timing Nocturnal / Diurnal
Have child ever dry for continuous 6 months
# of wet night/ week
Associated Sxs:

- Dysuria
- Frequency
- Urgency
- Hesitancy
- Polyuria / polydipsia
- Abnormal urine stream
- Low back pain
- Lower extremities weakness or paresthesia

Drinking Habits before bedtime
Sleeping pattern/snoring/ Sleep apnea
Hx of any problems with toilet training
Constipation / Encopresis
Home Environment changes/ other
Psychological Stressors
(e.g Divorce/ New baby/ changes in Home or school, death in family)
What is parents respond to bedwetting
Rewards or punishments used
Dry when sleep away from home
Any past medical investigations or Interventions & its effectiveness?

PMH: Hx of recurrent UTI, urological abnormalities

PSH: urological surgeries

Meds Hx: Diuretics, other medications

Allergy:

Family Hx: parent or siblings with Hx of enuresis

Social Hx: who lives with patient

PERTIENT PHYSICAL EXAM

Check vital signs & parametric measurements *(centiles)*

EYE: Fundus (papilledema)

ABD: Renal mass

GNEITAL: labial adhesions, FB, rectal tone, perianal sensation, anal wink

BACK: spinal defects, sacral dimple, hair tuft

NEURO: Lower extremities tone, reflexes, sensation, Babinski sign, gait

DIFFERENTIAL DIAGNOSIS

Primary Enuresis (Dx of exclusion)

Secondary Enuresis

- UTI
- Constipation
- Diabetes mellitus
- Diabetes insipidus
- Kidney disease
- Anatomic abnormalities of the urinary tract
- Sleep disorders
- Anxiety or behavioral disorders
- Medications *(sedatives, diuretics, antihistamines)*
- Diuretics, caffeine, (methylxanthines)
- Spinal cord disease

MENSTRUAL HISTORY

Age of menarche

LMP

Length of menstrual flow   # of bleeding days

Frequency

Cycle Regularity

Bleeding amount (heavy, average, light) # of pads used per day

Associated Cramps …..severity

Inter-menstrual Spotting

Hx of pregnancy/ abortion

Hx of abnormal pap smear

SEXUAL HISTORY

Sexually active?

Men/women interest

Type of contact (oral/ vaginal / anal)

Number of current partners

Number of Partners over last year

Use of protections

Use of contraception

Hx of STIs

VAGINAL DISCHARGE

Duration:
Discharge details

- Color
- Amount
- Consistency
- Odor

Course: worsening, Constant
Frequency intermittent, Static
Associated Sxs

- Genital itchiness
- Genital soreness
- Genital rash
- Dysuria
- Fever
- Dyspareunia
- Abnormal vag bleeding (*intermenstrual, post-coital*)
- Abdominal / Pelvic pain

Hx of vag. Foreign body
Ask about Menstrual & Sexual Hx (*see page 88*)

PMH: DM, recurrent UTI, PID, STI

PSH: any previous surgeries

Meds Hx:

Allergy:

Family Hx:

Social Hx: Smoking, alcohol or illicit drug abuse, recent travel, occupation

PENILE DISCHARGE

Duration:
Discharge Hx

- Color
- Amount
- Consistency
- Odor

Course: worsening, Constant
Associated Sxs

- Genital itchiness
- Genital soreness
- Genital rash
- Dysuria
- Fever
- Abdominal / Genital pain

Ask about Sexual Hx (*see page 88*)

PMH: DM, recurrent UTI, STIs

PSH: any previous surgeries

Meds Hx:

Allergy:

Family Hx:

Social Hx: Smoking, alcohol or illicit drug abuse, recent travel, occupation

AMENORRHEA

Duration
Did start menarche?

- <u>If not:</u> presence of secondary sexual characteristics? *Axillary hair, Pubic hair & breast*
- <u>If yes:</u> *when was* last period? And ask about Menstrual Hx *(see page 88)*

Sexual Hx: *(see page 88)*

Obstetric hx

- Possible current pregnancy
- Previous pregnancy/ Gravity/ Parity Last pregnancy
- Hx of post-partum Hemorrhage
- Hx of abortions
- Last pap smear

Recent life stressors
Recent change in exercise or eating habits

Associated Sxs

- Pelvic pain
- Acne
- Hirsutism
- Wt gain / Loss
- Cold / heat intolerance
- Palpitation
- Headache
- Loss of peripheral vision
- Galactorrhea
- Loss sense of smell
- Depressed mood
- Fatigue

Post-menopausal sxs

- Hot flashes
- Loss of libido
- Vaginal dryness
- Night sweats
- Mood changes

PMH:
Hx of any chronic diseases
Hx of thyroid disorders
PCOS
DM
Endometriosis
Hx of malignancy or radiation exposure

PSH:
Any pelvic surgeries
Hx of thyroid surgery

Meds Hx:

- Current meds
- Contraceptives
- Others: Antithyroid, Antipsychotic, Methyldopa, Chemotherapies

Allergy:

Family Hx:
Constitutional delayed puberty
FH of breast or pelvic tumors
FH of premature menopause

Social Hx:
Smoking, Alcohol, or illicit drug abuse

PERTIENT PHYSICAL EXAM

Check Parametric measures & BMI

GEN: Built, dysmorphism, short stature

NECK: webbed neck, thyroid exam

SKIN: Hirsutism, acne, acanthosis nigricans, stria

BREAST: tanner stage, Galactorrhea, wide nipple line *(Turner syndrome)*

ABD: abdominal masses (*tumor or pregnancy*)

GENITALIA: Tanner stage, pubic hair, ambiguous genitalia, clitoromegaly, Hymen

Ask permission for genital and speculum pelvic exam (if indicated)

DIFFERENTIAL DIAGNOSIS

Primary Amenorrhea (*no menarche by age of 15*)

- Turner Syndrome
- Pregnancy
- Constitutional
- Congenital adrenal hyperplasia
- Outflow obstruction (imperforated hymen, vaginal septum)
- Androgen insensitivity
- Prolactin secreting tumors
- Kallmann syndrome
- Thyroid disease
- Cushing syndrome

Secondary Amenorrhea

- Pregnancy
- Hypothalamic Pituitary pathology
- Pituitary adenomas (loss of negative feedback inhibition)
- Anorexia, Wt loss, aggressive exercise, stress (hypothalamic inhibition)
- Prolactin secreting tumors
- ACTH secreting tumors
- Hypothalamic infiltrates or tumors
- Empty-sella syndrome
- Sheehan syndrome
- Adrenal Pathology
- Non-classic adrenal hyperplasia
- Adrenal Tumors
- Ovarian pathology
- POCS
- Premature ovarian failure
- Acquired ovarian failure (cytotoxic drugs or radiation)
- Ovarian tumors
- Uterine adhesions
- Thyroid disease
- Cushing syndrome
- Drug-induced

ABNORMAL VAGINAL BLEEDING

Duration
Frequency
How long it lasts
Amount of bleeding: how many pads/hr
Passing clots?
Timing
Intermenstrual, post-menopausal, post coital
Bleeding from other body sites
Hx of vaginal trauma or FB
Menstrual Hx

- Last period
- Frequency: Regular or not
- Length of each cycle
- Bleeding amount
- Associated cramps or breast tenderness
- Age of Menarche
- Age of Menopause

Sexual Hx *(see page 88)*

Obstetric hx

- Hx of recent abortion or pregnancy
- Other Previous pregnancy/ Gravity/ Parity Last pregnancy
- Hx of complications
- Last pap smear

Associated Sxs

- Fever
- Abdominal/pelvic pain
- Vaginal discharge or itchiness
- Wt gain / Loss
- Cold / heat intolerance
- Palpitation
- Dizziness/ fainting

PMH: hx of easy bruising, chronic diseases

PSH: any previous surgeries

Meds Hx:
Current medications
Anticoagulant, ASA, hormonal therapy

Family Hx:
FH of bleeding disorders
FH of ovarian, uterine or breast cancers

Social Hx:
Smoking, alcohol, illicit drugs abuse

PERTIENT PHYSICAL EXAM

Check Parametric measures & BMI

GEN: Built, pallor, signs of distress

NECK: LAD, thyroid exam

SKIN: petechia or bruises, Hirsutism, acne, acanthosis nigricans, stria

ABD: abdominal masses (*tumor or pregnancy*)

Genitalia: external abrasions or discharge,

Ask permission for speculum pelvic exam (*if indicated*)

DIFFERENTIAL DIAGNOSIS

Localized Gynecological disorders
- Pregnancy
- Ectopic pregnancy
- Abortion
- Retained conception products
- Endometriosis
- Infections: cervicitis, endometritis
- Tumors: cervical/ uterine
- Trauma laceration, FB, …

Systemic disorders

- Thyroid disease, PCOS, Cushing syndrome
- Coagulopathy
- Thrombocytopenia / PLT dysfunction
- Medications side effects
- Renal or hepatic failures

ATAXIA

Duration
Do you feel weak or imbalanced?
Onset: sudden, gradual
Course: worsening, Constant
Frequency intermittent, Static
Previous episodes
Preceding seizures
Recent infection
Hx of head or lower extremities Trauma
Does it worse when you close your eyes
Associated Sxs

- Fever
- Rash
- Nausea/ vomiting
- Leg pain
- dizziness
- Hearing or visual problems
- Headache
- Weakness or numbness
- Seizures
- Incontinence
- Dementia

PMH:
Hx of head trauma
Hx of cardiovascular diseases (HTN, DM, Hyperlipidemia, stroke....
Hx of congenital heart disease *(stroke)*
Hx of brain neoplasms
Hx of malignancy (metastasis)
PSH:
Previous brain or spinal cord surgeries
Meds Hx:
Vaccination Hx: recent vaccination
Allergy:
Family Hx: Family members with ataxia

Social Hx:
Excess alcohol intake
Smoking, illicit drug abuse
Diet (vegan), Occupation

PERTINENT PHYSICAL EXAM

EYE: nystagmus, pupils, EOM, papilledema

EAR: Weber, Rinne tests

SKIN: neurofibromas, hemangiomas, telangiectasia

MSK: scoliosis, pes caves

Complete neuro exam: Tone, power, Reflexes, sensation, cranial nerves, Babinski sign, cerebellar signs and gait

Cerebellar sings: dysdiadochokinesia (*impaired rapid, alternating hand movements*), ataxia, nystagmus, intention tremor, scanning dysarthria, heel–shin test positive

DIFFERENTIAL DIAGNOSIS

- Postinfectious cerebellar ataxia
- Postictal
- Intoxication
- Posttraumatic
- Brain tumor
- Inner ear pathology
- Thiamine deficiency
- Migraine
- MS/ ADEM
- Guillain-Barre' syndrome
- Stroke
- Familial periodic ataxia: Family history
- Psychogenic
- Friedreich ataxia
- Ataxia telangiectasia

SEIZURE

When happened?
Type of seizures?

- Tonic clonic (shaking)
- Spastic (stiffness)
- Absent (stay still, staring & unresponsive)

How long it lasted?
Any previous episodes?
If not, when was the last episode? And how frequent they happen?
Factors for seizures such as sleep deprivation, alcohol ingestion, stress, fever
Hx of head trauma

Pre-ictal

- Aura
- Visual/ auditory hallucinations
- Light floaters

Ictal

- LOC
- Cyanosis
- Up rolling of eyes
- Tongue biting
- Bladder/bowel Incontinence

Post-ictal (*if any how long it lasted?*)

- Lethargy
- confusion
- Amnesia
- Aphasia
- Weakness of paralysis

Associated Sxs

- Headaches
- Early morning vomiting
- Fever
- Focal weakness

PMH: if has hx of epilepsy, when diagnosed? who diagnosed it? What was treatment? Last follow up.
Any other chronic medical conditions

PSH: any previous surgeries

Meds Hx: current medication, name, dose, recent medications or dose changes, treatment compliance

Vaccination Hx: recent vaccination

Allergy:
Family Hx: FH of seizure disorders

Social Hx: smoking, alcohol, illicit drugs abuse, sexual history, recent travel

---

Meningeal Signs

- **nuchal rigidity**

- **Brudzinski sign**: neck flexion on involuntary hip flexion

- **Kernig's sign:** hip flexed◻ knee extension cause pain

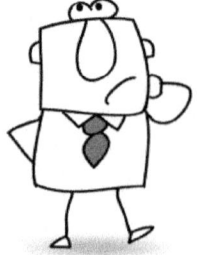

PERTIENT PHYSICAL EXAM

Check vital signs and O2 sat

ABC if still seizing

HEAD signs of trauma, macro or microcephaly, Bulging AF in infants

SKIN: look for neurocutaneous disorders manifestations (Café-au-lait spots, neurofibromas, facial angiofibroma, Unilateral port-wine facial nevus, ash leaf spots)

Complete neuro exam: GCS, alert, oriented, Tone, power, DT Reflexes, sensation, cranial nerves II- XII, Babinski sign, cerebellar signs and gait, Look for meningeal Signs

DIFFERENTIAL DIAGNOSIS

- Epilepsy
- CNS infection
- Brain tumors
- Stroke, AVM, brain hemorrhage
- Neurocutaneous disorders
- Intoxication/ Medications: amphetamines, …
- Anticonvulsant withdrawal

HEADACHE

Duration
Onset
Location
Character
Progression/Frequency
Lasts for….
Severity
Severe enough to wake up from sleep
Diurnal variation
Radiation
Aggravated by
- Stress
- Bright light
- Noise
- Bending forward *(sinusitis)*
- Touching scalp or chewing *(temporal neuritis)*

Relieved by
Analgesics
Dark quit place

Hx of head trauma

Associated sxs:

- Fever
- Aura
- Tearing/ Runny nose
- Retro-orbital pain
- Visual disturbance
- Facial pain
- Neck pain/ stiffness
- Early morning vomiting
- Speech difficulty
- Photophobia
- Phonophobia
- Extremity weakness
- Numbness/tingling
- Dizziness
- Gait Instability
- Rash

PMH: any chronic diseases

PSH: any previous surgeries

Medication: OCP use in female, chronic analgesia use (rebound headache), others

FH: Migraine, Brain Tumor

Social Hx: Recent stress, smoking, alcohol, caffeine, illicit drug abuse

PERTIENT PHYSICAL EXAM

Check vital signs

Perform complete PE with focus on neuro exam.

GCS, alert, oriented, Tone, power, DT Reflexes, sensation, cranial nerves II- XII, Babinski sign, cerebellar signs and gait, Look for meningeal Signs

DIFFERENTIAL DIAGNOSIS

Acute Headache

- CNS infection
- Upper respiratory infection
- Intracranial hemorrhage
- Venous sinus thrombosis
- VP shunt malfunction
- Post LP headache

Recurrent Non- Progressive Headache

- Tension headache
- Analgesic / Caffeine overuse (rebound headache)
- Migraine
- Cluster headache
- Sinusitis
- Hypertension
- AVM malformation
- Post-traumatic headache
- Temporomandibular joint syndrome
- Pseudotumor cerebri
- Temporal neuritis

Recurrent Progressive Headache
- Brain Tumor
- Hydrocephalus
- Lead poisoning
- Arnold-Chiari malformation (hydrocephalus)

MEMORY LOSS

Duration
Type: forget everything or some
Onset: sudden, gradual
Course: worsening, Constant
Time course worsen over days/ months/ years
Effect on daily activities
Hx of head trauma
Vegetarian diet *(vit B12 def.)*
Associated Sxs

- Speech difficulty
- Headache
- Weakness/ numbness
- Mood changes
- Personality changes
- Hallucinations
- Delusions
- Abnormal gait
- Urinary incontinence
- Cold/ heat intolerance
- Fatigue
- Wt gain/ loss

PMH:
Stork, TIA, hypertension, depression

PSH: any previous surgeries

Meds Hx:

Family Hx:
Dementia run in family esp. <65y

Social Hx:
alcohol intake, Smoking
Recent travel
Sexual Hx ($)
Occupation
Social support

PERTIENT PHYSICAL EXAM

Check Mini mental status:
Alertness/ Orientation

(ask about name, DOB, date of today)
Memory status

(memorize 3 words e.g. Car, Red, Flag)
Concentration

(spell WORLD forward & backward)
Judgement

(what to do if there is a fire in the trash ban)

Complete neuro exam: GCS, alert, oriented, Tone, power, DT Reflexes, sensation, cranial nerves II- XII, Babinski sign, cerebellar signs and gait, Look for meningeal Signs

DIFFERENTIAL DIAGNOSIS

- Depression or stress, sleep deprivation *(pseudodementia)*
- Vitamin B 12 deficiency
- Korsakoff dementia
- Post traumatic head injury
- Vascular dementia (stroke)
- Lewy body dementia
- Chronic subdural hematoma
- Normal pressure hydrocephalus
- Late neurosyphilis
- AIDS associated dementia
- Alzheimer's disease
- Delirium
- Hypothyroidism, hyperthyroidism

JOINT PAIN

Location
Duration:
Onset: sudden, gradual
Course: worsening, constant
Frequency: intermittent, Static
Radiation
Severity
Diurnal variation
Other joints involved
Previous episodes
Aggravating factors
Relieving factors
Hx of Trauma
Hx of tick bite
Associated Sxs

- Joint Swelling
- Fever
- Weight loss
- Morning stiffness
- Clicking, Locking, Limitation of motion
- Headache
- Fatigue
- Skin rash
- Chest pain, dyspnea
- Dysuria, hematuria
- Bloody diarrhea
- Red eyes,

PMH:

PSH:

Meds:

Family Hx: Similar sxs, Hx rheumatological dz

Social Hx: Recent travel,
Joint overuse / Occupation
Animal contact
intravenous drug abuse

LOW BACK PAIN

Location
Duration
Onset: sudden, gradual
Course: worsening, constant
Frequency: intermittent, static
Quality: sharp, dull, stretching, electrical
Radiation
Severity
Diurnal variation
Other joints involved
Previous episodes
Aggravating factors

- Certain position
- Prolonged standing
- Walking
- Coughing

Relieving factors

- Rest
- Exercise
- Pain meds

Hx of Trauma
Associated Sxs

- Fever
- Night sweats, Wt loss
- Morning stiffness
- Urine or stool incontinence
- Perianal numbness
- Lower extremities weakness
- Abdominal pain
- Nausea/ vomiting
- Related to menstrual cycle

PMH: Malignancy, any chronic medical illness
PSH: any previous surgeries
Meds Hx: current medication
Family Hx: Arthritis, Autoimmune diseases

Social Hx: Smoking, alcohol, IV drug abuse, occupation

PERTIENT PHYSICAL EXAM

GEN: built, posture, signs of distress due to pain

ABD: abdominal masses, (spinal cord compression) saddle anesthesia, anal wink, rectal tone

SKIN: café-au-lait spots

BACK: inspec for sacral dimple, sacral lipoma, hair tuft, deformities or signs of trauma

point tenderness over spines & sacroiliac joint or paraspinal muscle tenderness.

Back ROM flexion, extension, lateral bending & rotation.

NEURO complete exam with more focus on lower extremities including gait.

DIFFERENTIAL DIAGNOSIS

- Trauma, muscle spasm
- Disc herniation
- Spinal canal stenosis
- Osteoarthritis
- Compression fracture
- Ankylosing spondylitis
- Epidural abscess
- Osteomyelitis
- Discitis
- Spinal cord compression by neoplasm or metastasis
- Referred visceral pain: renal colic, endometriosis, pelvic inflammatory disease, abdominal aortic aneurysm

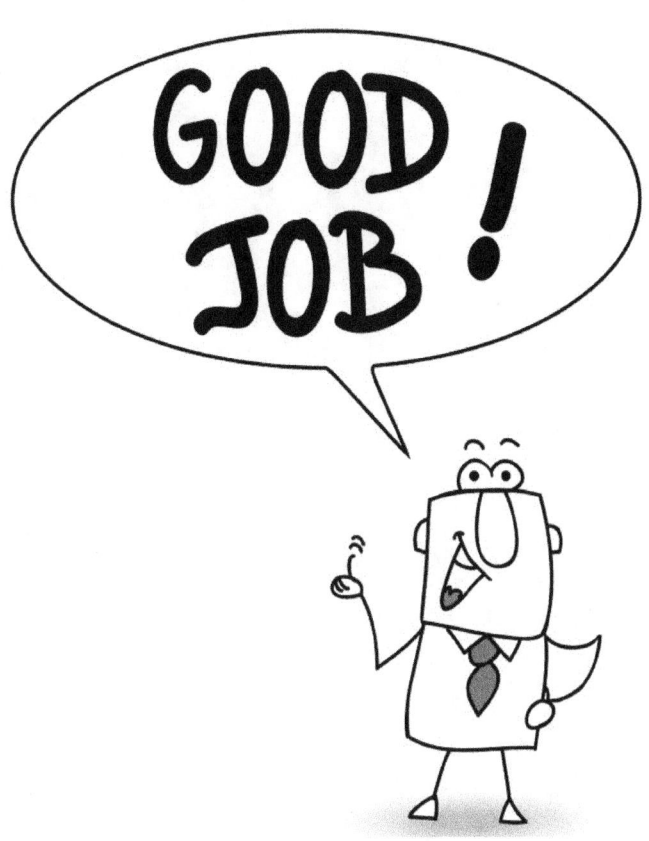

www.ingramcontent.com/pod-product-compliance
Lightning Source LLC
Chambersburg PA
CBHW070657220526
45466CB00001B/476